Managing Migraines

By
Sally White

ISBN-13:978-1494311445
ISBN-10:1494311445

Content

Foreword

Migraine has become a dreaded word for the thousands of sufferers all over the world. It is a disease that can put you out of action for a couple of hours or for a couple of days. Because of this it has an enormous effect on the economies of the world. There is no definite cure for these debilitating headaches and science has not yet proved what the exact cause is.

I have made a study of the remedies and realise that unless you want to become a victim of the "cure" as well, you need to start becoming pro active and investigate for yourself what it is that triggers off your attacks.

It is no good taking drugs to get relief from pain and with each attack you require stronger drugs. In the end the drugs will be just such a problem as the migraine. By taking authority over your condition you can start keeping a diary of the events just before the attack started. Write down what you ate that day, how you felt emotionally just before the headache started, were you over tired, stressed, or angered.

With time you will have a pattern of events and you will be able to see which emotions contributed to your attack. You will be able to sense which types of food you eat that seem to trigger off an attack. With this information in hand you can then begin to eliminate food types one at a time and see if there is any improvement in your condition. This might be a slow process, but it will be a sure way and you will be able to control your well being without turning constantly to chemical substances for relief of pain.

After watching immediate family members suffer for years from this disease I decided to do something to help them. This system is slow but sure and in most cases it will bring positive results to the sufferer.

For the many sufferers who have their attacks brought on by motion sickness it is a good idea to only take short journeys at a time. If you have to go on a long journey break it up and have rest periods often so that you do not begin to feel nauseous. I have included various medications that a doctor can prescribe for you if you really need instant relief. There are medications that can be taken to ward off attacks. If you do need to make use of them while you are investigating your pattern of attacks that is fine as long as you do not become dependant on them and lose sight of your goal to control the disease yourself.

I hope that the information I have gathered together will be beneficial to you and that you will find that by being pro active you are more in control of your disease.

Migraine

The word 'migraine' is French and is derived from the Greek word "hemicrania". Which means "half the head". This is a description of a migraine.

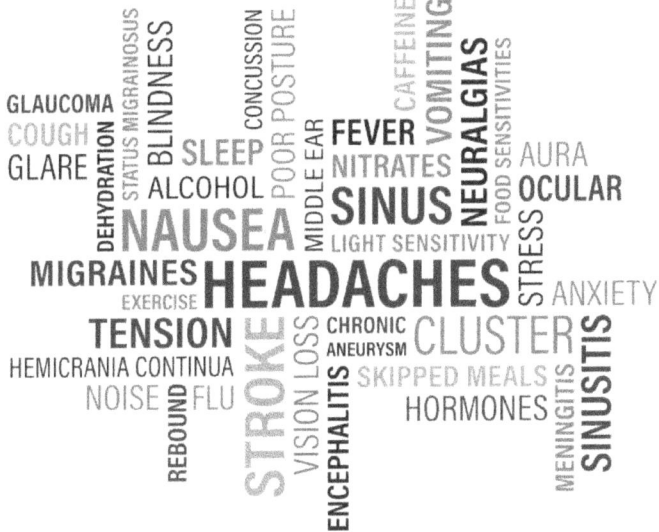

According to ancient records migraine is a disease that has been around for centuries. It can be traced way back to ancient Syria. There are ancient documents describing the symptoms and the cures they used to use. This seems to put a question mark on whether or not stress is one of the causes of attack. On the other hand we do not know what type of stress the ancient world had to deal with.

It almost always only attacks half the head at a time. This does not necessarily mean that it will be the same side every time you experience an attack. Quite often the front of the head is affected.

Migraine is a headache that can become disabling and it can occur frequently of less frequent depending on the severity of the disease.

This is a common neurological disease, which unfortunately many people suffer from. It is a very severe headache and as I stated it usually only attacks one side at a time. This is good fortune with the bad fortune. Otherwise the pain could become totally unbearable.

The fact that it does not necessarily always attack the same side of the head is also a mystery. These attacks can last from a few hours to a couple of days depending on the verity of the attack.

There are a number of symptoms one can experience as a result of this disorder, the main one being an excruciating headache. Dizziness and nausea accompanied by vomiting are also common symptoms.

In many cases the eyes are affected and the sufferer could experience partial blindness for a short time. Hearing could also be affected.

Sometimes sufferers will experience vagueness in their minds after an attack has subsided. There are many different symptoms that people report having. It appears that the symptoms depend on the severity of the attack experienced.

When groups of sufferers were asked about their symptoms it appeared that most of them experienced the same type of feeling. There were some participants of the study that suffered more symptoms than the rest of them or experienced them in a more intense way.

Sufferers experience various time spans between attacks. Many people have frequent attacks while others might have long periods between attacks. There could be gaps of weeks, months or even years between attacks. Many people will only ever experience one attack in a lifetime.

In many cases where young people are sufferers they eventually stop getting attacks once they get older. This is indeed a fortunate state of affairs.

Not all severe headaches are migraine there could possibly be another cause for the pain. Sufferers of headaches should check with their medical practitioners and not just assume that they have migraine.

They need to make sure that there is no other possible cause for the headache. It could be something that can be cured. It is better to have a medical examination rather than just diagnose the disease yourself.

There are two main types of migraine

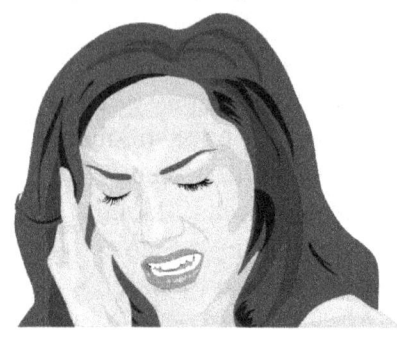

Migraine with aura (experiencing warning symptoms before an attack)

Migraine without aura (no warning symptoms experienced)

Migraine With Aura

This type of migraine is known as the classic sort.

An aura means that the migraine sufferer will experience a sensory warning sign about 10- 30 minutes before the headache actually sets in. The usual signs are the feeling of nausea and/or an aversion to bright lights and loud noises. You might see flashes of light before your eyes. Dizziness could set in and you could feel nauseous and vomit.

You could get blurred vision and partial deafness. Vision can be partly and temporarily lost while a feeling of numbness will take over the hands and arms this would feel like "pins and needles". This numbness could affect the face as well. Usually this numbness will be most acute in the lips and tongue.

Once the headache sets in these symptoms normally go away and the sufferer is left only with the acute headache. Many regular sufferers just have a feeling that there is a migraine on the way. It is usually a restless tired feeling.

There could be a mood swing as well that triggers a warning. After experiencing the feeling many times they will know how to identify it.

A bright light that suddenly shines in your eyes, even if it is just for a split second, can trigger off an attack in some sufferers or a very loud noise.

This type of migraine is more severe than the one without aura.

Migraine Without Aura

This type of migraine is known as the common sort.

These headaches start without any warning symptoms. They can start at any time of the day or night. One minute you will be feeling fine and the next you will be experiencing the pain of an attack.

It could just start as a dull throbbing, which is bearable or it could crescendo into a more aggressive pain.

There are times when the sufferer experiences unbearable pain that prevents them from being able to do anything except lay still on the bed in a darkened room until the pain subsides.

Almost always the patient has partial blindness from the pain and any form of concentration is virtually impossible. Noise of any kind makes the condition worse.

Usually this condition does not clear up until the patient has had a bout of vomiting. This seems to relieve the pressure in the head. The headache will then subside. This will not be the case with every attack.

Some attacks will last longer than others. They could last a few minutes or hours depending on the severity of the attack

Some sufferers are left feeling weak and listless for days after an attack. There could be a lack of concentration and a stiff neck.

If the symptoms are only visual and there are no other symptoms such as a headache consult an ophthalmologist in case the cause is an eye disease and not migraine. You could then get this condition treated.

Abdominal Migraine

Abdominal migraine is a condition that mainly occurs in children. They experience pain in the central abdominal area. They normally experience nausea and vomiting as well as loss of appetite. Many children suffer excessive nausea and vomiting but will not have a headache.

These attacks can last up to seventy-two hours at a time. Children will need to be kept comfortable, as they do not always understand what is going on in their bodies.

It is most likely that children who suffer from this type of migraine will begin to get migraine headaches, as they grow older. They do tend to become less again once they are adults. This is a least a good thing.

Fortunately there are many drugs that doctors have access to for children to help relieve their pain and make them comfortable.

It is good to check the child's diet and make sure that nothing is being eaten that could possibly trigger off an attack. Call in the help of a dietician if you are not sure what would be the best diet for a child of the relevant age.

Investigate if there are any outside factors that could trigger off an attack. Over excitement, any type of stress or fear. Make a note of the circumstances before an attack starts and what the patient has eaten and you could see a pattern in the attacks. By doing this you could be a great help in alleviating your child's pain.

There are a number of less know types of migraine namely

- Basilar artery migraine
- Headache free migraine
- Status migraine
- Ophthalmoplegic migraine
- Carotidynia

Basilar artery migraine is some sort of a disturbance of the major brain artery, which is situated at the base of the brain.

This type of migraine mostly attacks young women and is associated with the menstrual cycle. There are various symptoms, which include double vision and poor muscular coordination.

Headache free migraine has all the symptoms of the usual migraine except that there is no headache.

Status migraine is considered to be one of severest types of migraine as the pain is so intense that the sufferer in most cases has to be hospitalised. It usually lasts for more than 72 hours. Many patients have reported being depressed and anxious before an attack.

An Ophthalmoplegic migraine is when the sufferer has problems with their vision. It could be manifested as double vision or a droopy eyelid or other visual problems.

A carotidynia migraine is referred to as the facial migraine or the lower half headache. The reason for this is that the pain is a deep ache or sometimes a piercing pain in the neck and jaw. This can cause swelling over the carotid artery in the neck.

It seems to attack older people more often than younger ones. These attacks can occur several times a week and last from a few minutes to hours.

You can discuss these types of migraine with your medical practitioner if you have been diagnosed as suffering from one of them.

General Symptoms In Order To Identify Migraine

There are various symptoms, which can warn the sufferer that an attack is imminent.

It could start any time of the day or night. The pain might only be moderate or it could be very severe and of a throbbing nature.

It will become more intense as time goes on. It will eventually begin to ease off once it has reached its peak. The pain is usually on one side of the head but could be on both sides and in front depending on how severe the attack is.

Common symptoms are the feeling of nausea, vomiting, blurred vision and possibly the feeling of wanting to be alone in a dark room as light will be painful to the eyes.

Dizziness, tiredness, and in some cases retention of fluids could all be symptoms of an attack.

A throbbing headache is experienced which is often aggravated by anything that brings involuntary movement to the head. This feeling could wake one up during the night and could possibly last for many hours. It will leave the sufferer feeling weak and tired. It saps all the energy out of the sufferer.

Diarrhoea could also be a symptom especially in the case of children as they would be more inclined to have abdominal pain than head pain when they suffer from migraine.

When Should One Consult A Medical Practitioner?

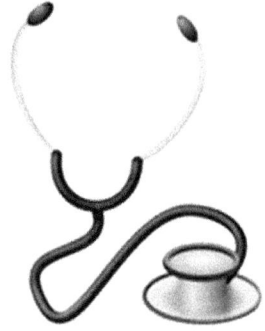

If the symptoms become too acute and the usual painkillers are not effective any more it is a good idea to consult with your doctor for advice.

If the pattern of your headache as you know it suddenly changes or it becomes more intense call your doctor immediately for advice.

If you find that you are having too frequent attacks and they are disrupting your life style you will need to pay the doctor a visit for further examinations or a change in prescription drugs.

You might find that the headache is always in the same place, which could indicate that it could possibly be something other than migraine.

Usually migraine is just on one side of the head but it does change sides and does occur in the front of the head as well.

If your headache gets worse when you lay down, call the doctor. You might be getting symptoms that you do not usually get. It would be safer to have the medical practitioner check them out to give you peace of mind. Your previously prescribed medication may suddenly not be effective anymore this would be a reason to call the doctor.

You might have bad side effects from medication and need advice from the physician. Watch out for irregular heartbeat, difficulty in staying awake, over fatigue, nausea and vomiting with diarrhoea and many other symptoms that you will feel are not normal. Call the doctor immediately so that he or she can change your medication.

Remember that your qualified medical practitioner is there to help and advise you so make the most of his expertise and call him when necessary.

Before you consult your doctor make a list of observations you have made in connection with your migraine attacks. Mention frequency of attacks, how often you miss time at work, how effective or ineffective your current medication is, do you have frequent nausea and vomiting attacks.

All these factors will make it easier for your doctor to assess your case and prescribe the correct medication for you.

Possible Causes Of Migraine

The cause of the pain has not definitely been pinpointed to any factor, but research has shown that blood vessels in some parts of the brain can go into a spasm. This would account for the aura. When the blood vessels dilate after this spasm, and then return to normal again, could be the cause of the severe pain.

More and more medical practitioners are coming to the conclusion that this is not a disease of the blood vessels but is primarily neurological as many sufferers report a sore tenderness in the area where the pain was. This can last a few days after the attack.

Some others report a sense of lack of concentration for days after a bad attack of migraine. This would point to it being neurological.

This side effect cannot be caused by blood vessels going into a spasm. Research is constantly on the go so there is sure to be more light thrown on the subject in the near future. At some stage the medical world thought this disease to be more an emotional disease but research is beginning to reveal that it is a neurological disease.

Some researchers think these headaches could be brought on by increased activity of certain chemicals in the brain. This would bring us to the question of what triggers off this increased activity of chemicals?

There is the possibility of genes playing a part and that would then make you more prone to being a sufferer of migraine.

This has not been proven but there is a growing understanding of genetic causes and this could be a breakthrough in the near future.

There are many cases were a couple of members of one family suffer from this disease which does seen to point to the fact that genetics could have an influence on the sufferers.

Most doctors believe that migraine is caused by stress in one form or another or something in the diet could trigger it off.

Dairy products, caffeine, red wine, chocolate and citrus fruits are some of the foods that are thought to be culprits.

Many people suffer migraine as a result of glaring or flickering lights or very loud noises. Anxiety and stress of any sort or becoming over tired can all be factors that contribute to an attack.

Change in the hormones in women during menopause and of those just before the commencement of their menstrual cycle could also be the cause of triggering off these debilitating headaches.

Many women find that these headaches disappear during pregnancy, while others only start having headaches when they are pregnant.

Many women taking oral contraceptives also experience migraine attacks. It might be a good idea to keep a record of your menstrual cycles and at what stage a headache sets in. After a couple of months you could possibly discover whether your attacks are indeed induced by your menstrual cycle or not.

There are many women who are only affected by headaches when they reach menopause. Research has not revealed what these natural hormones have to do with migraine.

There is a school of thought that is of the opinion that migraine can be linked to estrogen levels in a woman. As the estrogen level drops before a woman has her period this could trigger off migraine in some women. Women who suffer from this type of menstrual migraine report that these migraine attacks last longer than any other type. They can last up to seventy-two hours at a time and be very severe.

More often you experience nausea and vomiting at this time of the month. It also seems more difficult to treat these attacks than at a different time of the month.

During pregnancy when estrogen levels is high less women experience migraine. There is no proof that this is the case but it does seem to indicate that there is some truth in it.

The sufferer can help themselves by trying to discover what substance is causing the migraine. You would have to go through a process of elimination to discover exactly which substance or circumstance was causing the attack.

You would have to discuss your theories with your doctor and together you could find a way of eliminating certain factors from your lifestyle.

Up to 50% of migraine sufferers will also suffer from motion sickness. This is a very interesting fact as it does make researches realise that they need to understand the part motion sickness plays in migraine sufferers.

It could be that motion sets off some over activity in the chemicals of the brain. By investigating this fact they could possibly improve their understanding of the physiology of both problems.

Because patients have such varied symptoms it is a very difficult disease to treat. They do not always experience the same symptoms with every attack. This is why it is so important for sufferers of migraine to start taking note of what happens just before an attack occurs.

What mental state you were in and what you had to eat are of vital importance. If you keep a note of this you will probably be able to see a pattern emerging and this will make it so much easier to prevent these attacks in the first place.

Depression could also be a factor that could trigger off migraine attacks. This is a disease the affects most aspects of your life and affects the people you live with. When you are experiencing an attack it puts pressure on your immediate family.

It could be that family outings or family times together are disrupted while you have to work through the debilitating pain. This is no fault of the sufferer and the family has to learn to handle the situation.

Diagnosis

It is very difficult to diagnose migraine, as there is not enough information on the subject. When a patient has frequent severe headaches, doctors normally conclude that you are a migraine sufferer when they have asked numerous questions about the type of pain you suffer.

They find by asking questions about your attacks they can find out more about your condition than they would from a physical examination.

They will want to know about your work situation, your sleep pattern and also about previous injuries to your head and/or eyes. There are various factors that could point to another cause being responsible for the headache.

They will ask about your general health and examine you to make sure that there can be no other cause for the headaches.

If the medical practitioners find it necessary they will let you undergo a CT (computed tomographic) scan or an EEG (electroencephalogram) to make sure that there is no injury to the brain that could possibly be causing the pain. They might do a MRI (spinal tap scan) and a MRA (magnetic resonance angiography) if they think that is necessary.

These tests are necessary as the headaches could be caused by various other factors such as dilated blood vessels or bleeding in the brain. There are a number of reasons that could cause headaches.

When all these tests have been done and there is no visible damage detected to the brain they will safely be able to conclude that you are indeed a migraine sufferer.

Remember that there are no symptoms between attacks. There is no physical evidence that you can show a medical practitioner. You must visit your health carer while you are suffering an attack or just after you have had one when there is still physical evidence of the attack. Swollen eyes, stiff neck and so on.

Prevention

It is a good idea to gather as much information as you can about migraine if you are prone to these attacks. The more knowledge you have the easier it will be to understand what is causing the pain and this in turn will make it easier to manage it.

The National Institute of Neurological Disorders and Stroke is constantly doing research to get a better understanding of the disease and to improve on treatment. It is a good thing to know that there is ongoing research to find out more about this disease. Only by doing research will they eventually be able to come up with a proper diagnosis and the best cures for sufferers.

Prevention is always better than cure. As soon as you feel the first symptom of an oncoming attack, take a painkiller. This will prevent the pain from becoming too severe later on.

Get your doctor to prescribe an anti migraine drug. This will prevent migraine altogether or it will prevent the pain becoming too intense later on. Once migraine has set in it will take its course and it will be very difficult to break the pattern of pain later on.

It can be very helpful to take aspirin or paracetamol or similar painkillers and rest in a darkened room until you feel the symptoms subside. A quiet darkened room does a lot to ease the throbbing. Apply a cold compress to the head. This can also be very advantageous to relieve the throbbing pain.

A relaxing bath or shower can also prove to be advantageous to de stress yourself.

Swimming or taking regular walks also tends to reduce the frequency of attacks. This comes back to regular exercise and living a healthy lifestyle.

If you normally suffer from nausea along with all the other symptoms it would be a good idea to get a drug from your doctor that would counteract both symptoms at the same time.

If you are a frequent sufferer it might be a good idea to get your general practitioner to prescribe something for you that will give you relief before the headache becomes too bad. Many people believe in just laying in a darkened room and waiting until the symptoms wear off. This could take very long in certain instances.

It is far better to treat the pain as soon as possible. Why suffer if you do not have to? There are many modern migraine treatments that you might not be aware of that your doctor could prescribe for you. Anti migraine drugs taken before the headache gets started will be very helpful in preventing the headache from being very severe.

If you are a chronic sufferer of migraine your doctor could prescribe something for you to take daily which would prevent you from having so many attacks. It would probably not stop the attacks completely but will be a deterrent to a certain extent.

As with most other drugs anti migraine drugs can also have adverse side effects. The wisest course of action is to take them under supervision of your medical practitioner so that he can monitor your reaction to them.

Report any side effects to your medical practitioner immediately.

If stress is triggering off your headache attacks it could be very advantageous to learn to relax and to be able to control your feelings of anxiety

By learning to handle and avoid stress you could save yourself going through these regular debilitating attacks.

It is a good idea to take relaxation classes and learn how to totally relax every limb. You will be amazed how much better this can make you feel. It is well worth the time and effort spent.

Researchers are beginning to associate migraine with an increased risk of strokes in women. Women, who suffer from migraine, take oral contraceptives and smoke are putting themselves at a high risk of getting a stroke.

They are not advocating that you should stop taking oral contraceptives, but are advising women to stop smoking as soon as possible.

It might be a good idea to use some other form of contraceptives if you have close relatives who have heart disease or suffer from strokes. You might find that this is your answer to alleviating your migraine attacks. This is a matter, which you must discuss with your doctor.

It is always good to investigate all possibilities when you are trying to find out

what triggers off your attacks. This disease can change your lifestyle for the worse and it is worth every effort to investigate every avenue in order to rid yourself of the disease or lessen the attacks to some degree.

Natural Remedies

Before discussing natural remedies such as herbs it is always good to remember that herbs, as with drugs can have side effects, which can be mild or more dangerous.

One should especially be aware of drugs imported from Asia. Many of these drugs contain substances that could be detrimental to your health in their raw form. They could have bad side effects and could even cause death.

It is always wise to purchase these herbs from legal health stores where they have been correctly processed and labelled. The dosage per age will be clearly defined and side effects will be noted. Adhere to the instructions and they will be safe to take.

Exercise extreme caution before taking herbal remedies. Rather consult a medical practitioner and make sure that they are safe. Side effects could be very unpleasant.

Herbs Feverfew (Tanacetum Pantheism)

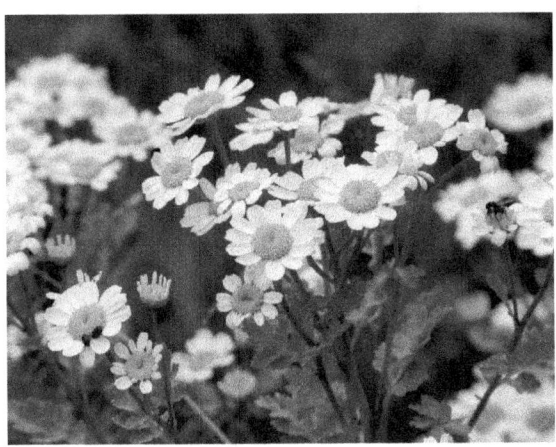

These herbs have been used for centuries to relieve the excruciating pain of migraine and various other pains. It is effective in most cases. There have been studies made on this herb.

Unfortunately there are many side effects of this herb and should not be taken without consulting a medical doctor or qualified healthcare practitioner.

They should not be taken by pregnant women or women hoping to become pregnant as it is not know what the effect on them will be.

Butterbur (Petasites Hybridus)

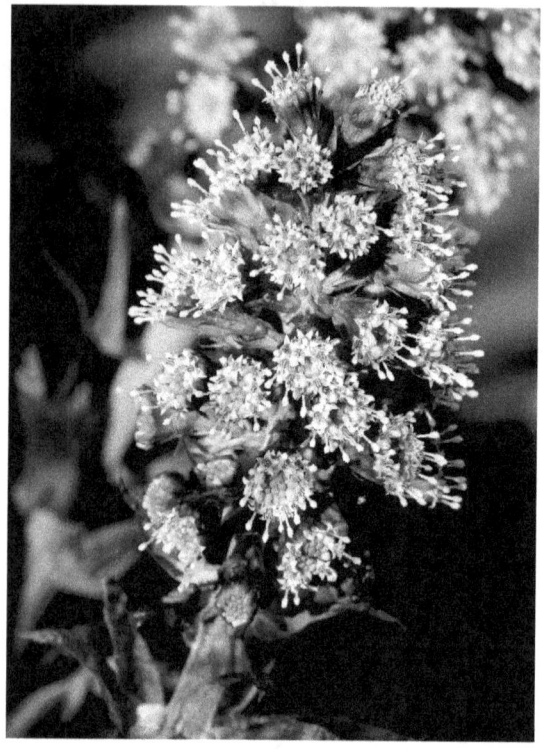

Tests done by researchers using this substance on migraine sufferers, seems to indicate that it does help prevent attacks. It is derived from a plant found in parts of northern Asia, areas in North America and in Europe.

Tests were done on migraine patients and it was found that a few milligrams of this substance twice a day were very effective in migraine sufferers. As with all herbs and drugs there can be people that will suffer from side effects.

It could induce vomiting and diarrhoea or alternatively constipation and a feeling of extreme fatigue.

This herb is not only used in the treatment of migraine but also for certain allergies and coughs as well as stomach cramps.

It is not advisable to take the raw herb as it contains pyrrolizidine alkaloids. They are extremely toxic to kidneys and liver and could cause serious allergies or worse still, cancer.

It is better to buy the product over the counter in a processed and diluted form. Read the label carefully and take the dosage as prescribed. Overdosing can be dangerous.

Coenzyme Q10

A study showed that sufferers who took this substance for a period of three months reported a reduction of headaches. It is a natural substance that is important for the transport of electrons. This substance has not been reported to have bad side effects. It is always advisable to first speak to your medical practitioner before you try any new substance to make sure that it will be right for you.

Phytoestorgens

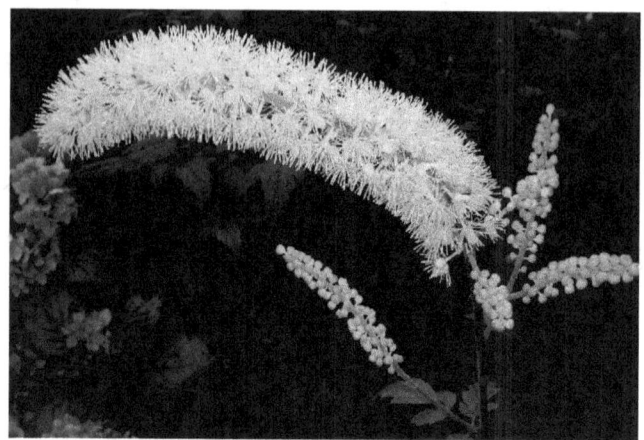

Black Cohosh

These are plant substances that have properties similar to estrogen. The plant products included are black cohosh and soy. These remedies should not be taken without consulting a qualified medical practitioner.

Magnesium

This has been found to be effective in the treatment of migraine. This is a mineral that is required for many functions of the body. It makes sense to

assume that a lack of the mineral could cause a condition like migraine. This has not definitely been proven to be a fact.

It is needed by the body for nerve functions, heart rhythm and blood pressure, the immune system, and for general bone health. It also helps with the regulation of blood sugar levels.

As can be seen this substance has many functions so it is not difficult to believe that it could be beneficial in the control of migraine.

It is particularly effective for patients who suffer from menstrual migraines who have a deficiency of this substance.

This mineral can be found in whole grains, nuts and seeds and green leafy vegetables. It is also obtainable in the form of a supplement from any health store.

As with all substances there can be side effects and these should be watched out for. Never overdose on any substance as this could create problems for you.

Side effects to watch out for are low blood pressure with irregular heart rate, diarrhoea and nausea, which in turn will cause loss of appetite.

Vitamin B2 (Riboflavin)

This vitamin is also believed to be advantageous for migraine sufferers. It is generally safe and there are reports of sufferers benefiting by it. it is obtainable in supplement form from any health store.

Overdosing can cause diarrhoea in some people so read the label carefully and adhere to the recommended dosage.

Kudzu Root (Pueraria Libata)

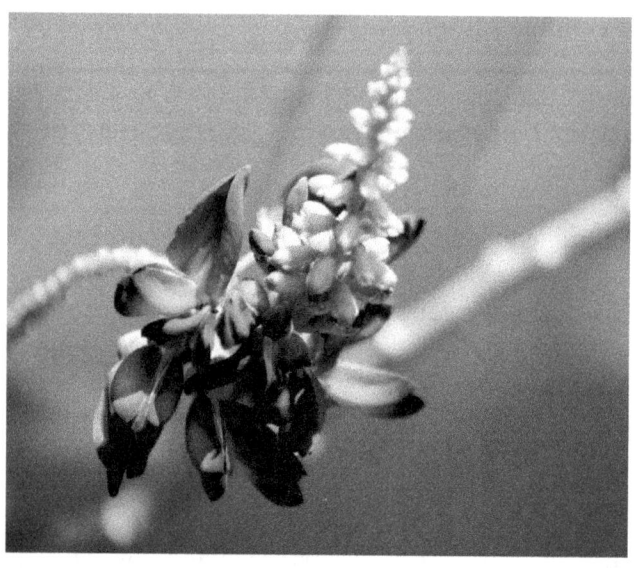

This substance has an effect on the serotonin receptors and is a great help in alleviating pain in menstrual migraine sufferers.

Fish Oil

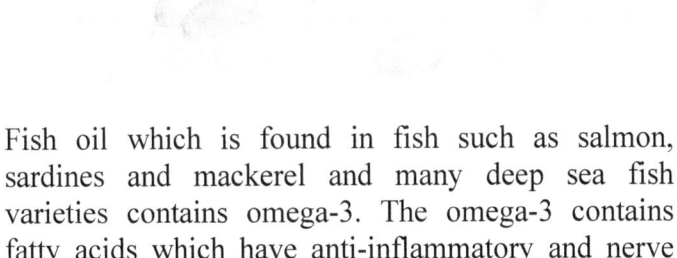

Fish oil which is found in fish such as salmon, sardines and mackerel and many deep sea fish varieties contains omega-3. The omega-3 contains fatty acids which have anti-inflammatory and nerve protecting properties which could be beneficial for migraine sufferers.

They are freely available in supplement form from any health store. They are not only beneficial for this complaint but are excellent for the general well being of the body.

The Use Of Drugs to Alleviate Pain

The use of drugs is not always recommended unless the pain becomes unbearable. If it is possible it will be far better to control what is causing the migraine and in this way minimise the amount of attacks you have.

By taking a shower or bath and bathing your head can bring many people relief. Resting in a dark room where everything is quiet is also very advantageous.

Although caffeine is said to be a culprit for causing migraine a cup of coffee right at the beginning stages of the headache could help ward it off.

There are times of course that the pain can become too much to bear and one will grab at any straw to get relief. When the headache starts it is advisable then to immediately take aspirin or paracetomol to break the pattern of pain.

Drug treatment can either prevent the attack or alleviate the symptoms once they have already started.

Delaying this can cause the headache to last longer as once the pain has set in it is very difficult to break the pattern. The headache could last for hours or days.

During an attack the emptying of the stomach slows down and this results in the patient suffering from nausea and vomiting. Here aspirin combined with caffeine can be very effective.

There are many severe drugs on the market and should be taken with discretion. Only take drugs that you have discussed with your medical practitioner.

There are many other drugs among them being narcotic pain killers which will provide relief but do have unpleasant side effects.

Take them under supervision of your medical practitioner so they you do not open yourself to addiction. You do not want to add another problem to the one you already have.

There are preventive drugs which medical practitioners can prescribe. Many sufferers report that the dosage is inefficient to alleviate the pain. They are either not effective at all or they are not effective enough.

Many over the counter drugs are not effective enough if the pain is severe. Many sufferers can not afford to pay for triptans so physicians will have to prescribe something else.

You will have to keep going back to your physician until he can come up with something that does help you.

Be careful of certain drugs that you do not get addicted to them. Always discuss this factor with the physician.

Be Health Conscious

It is advisable to enjoy a healthy diet everyday. This could be very beneficial for the body as a whole and could be the factor to reduce migraine attacks. Get a dietician to recommend a good diet for you.

By avoiding fatty foods and reducing your intake of sugar you could reduce the onset of nausea. It could be that many migraine sufferers trigger off an attack when they become nauseous.

Eating regularly is a very important factor as well. By allowing your blood sugar to become too low you could trigger off an attack. It is a good idea to always have something with you to eat if you know that you will be away from home for a length of time and will not be in reach of eating facilities.

Dehydration can be a very important factor in triggering off an attack. Watch out for this and make sure you take in enough liquids.

By always being aware of your problem you can counteract the causes that you have pinpointed for triggering off an attack.

Exercising is so important for a healthy body. You might find that when the blood is flowing freely through your body and your heart beat has been stimulated by the exercise that you will feel good and you will certainly be more relaxed.

Very strenuous sport could be bad for you as many sufferers find that a sudden bump can trigger off an attack. Stick to the "gentler" sports and exercise without exposing yourself to the possibility of triggering off an attack with something that is too strenuous. A sudden jerk is enough to set off the cycle of migraine.

A good night's rest is also very important. This alleviates stress and leaves you feeling refreshed and relaxed in the morning and you will have less chance of getting a sudden attack.

Many sufferers get attacks of migraine when they allow themselves to become over tired.

It is a very good idea to take food supplements. Sometimes when you are very busy it is a natural tendency to eat food that is not high in nutritional value. By taking food supplements you make up for the loss.

Children suffering from migraine should also be put on a healthy diet. Try his for a while to see if there is any improvement before starting them on drug treatment.

Other Treatments

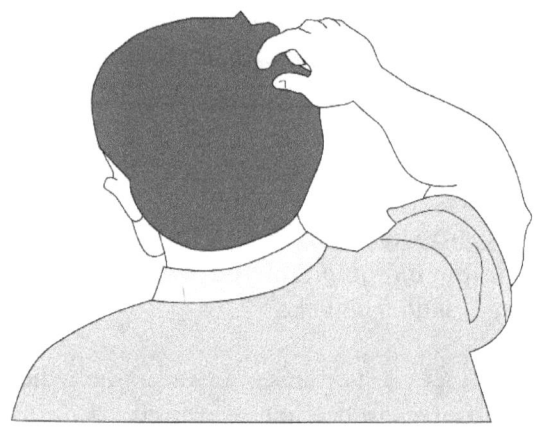

By Far The Best Treatment Is Prevention

Try and avoid any situation that you believe to be triggering off your attacks. If the migraine attacks are being triggered off by diet it is best to eliminate these foods from the diet. If you are not sure what exactly is triggering off your attacks, start eliminating suspect foods one at a time.

When you are sure that the eliminated food type is not the culprit you can re introduce it back into your diet again. You will with time be able to pinpoint which food substance it is that is the culprit.

It might not just be one food type but could be a combination of things. It could be a whole group of food. For instance, if cheese is causing the attacks you can be sure that all dairy products will be having some negative effect on you, in a lesser or greater degree.

Many sufferers find that ice cream triggers off the attacks and this will be traced back to the dairy product in the ice cream.

If stress is the culprit, try changing your lifestyle so that you will have the minimum amount of stress to cope with.

It would be a good idea to take up some form of relaxation classes where you have to train your mind to relax. You will be taught to relax your muscles and to teach your mind to switch off the daily hassles of life.

Try going for massage therapy. This could be very beneficial. As migraine sufferers could be prone to strokes it is very advisable to have as little stress to cope with as possible.

Massage therapy is a very good option as it will get rid of the stress particularly in your neck muscles that you are sometimes unaware of. After many attacks of migraine you can be left with a stiff neck and not be totally aware of it. This treatment will not only be effective in the reduction of attacks but could be the solution to stopping the attacks from occurring altogether. This could greatly improve your quality of life.

There are sufferers who find smelling certain substances to be beneficial when they feel the onslaught of an attack. One such substance is lavender.

You might want to speak to someone with the knowledge of plants at a health shop who could advise you which plants have a potent smell that could possibly give you relief when you feel the symptoms of the headache coming on.

Some sufferers find relief from smelling incense while others find that it aggravates the headache.

This will probably not cure the headache but could bring relief in the beginning stages.

Magnets

Many migraine sufferers find it very beneficial to alleviate pain by using magnets on the painful area of the head. If the pain is not too severe, this can be very beneficial in easing the pain. It is far better than making use of drugs to get relief from the pain.

These medical magnets are obtainable from medical stores. They do not claim to cure pain but only to bring comfort and to bring the pain to a tolerable level.

Acupuncture

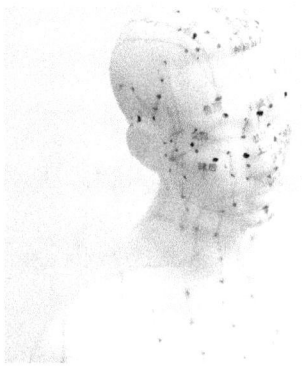

This ancient form of pain relief might help some sufferers. This is entirely up to you if you would like to try it or not. It could be beneficial in controlling the pain or pinpointing the problem. There have not been many reports that this form of treatment benefits sufferers of migraine.

Chiropractic

Your headaches could be caused by a vertebrae being out of alignment or some bone out of place. You could investigate this avenue by paying a visit to a chiropractor. He or she would be able to tell you if this is the case or not. They could treat you if this is the case. This could be the cure that you have been looking for.

As I have said before, when one is looking for a cure for this debilitating disease that can occur at any time and disrupt your life it is worth your while to explore every avenue in order to discover what is causing your problem.

Every problem has a cause and if we can only find out what the cause is we can solve the problem.

Not every migraine sufferer is going to be able to find out exactly what triggers off their attacks, but many will be able to find the cause and be relieved of this problem.

Applying Pressure

Many sufferers of migraine find that by applying pressure to the sore area with their thumb and index finger they can alleviate the pain especially in the beginning stages of the attack.

Abortive Treatment

Migraine sufferers will eventually learn to find their own way of coping with the pain in the beginning stages of the attack by aborting the symptoms before they get severe.

Cold or hot showers or baths depending on the individual will make a difference. Silence is a great soother accompanied by darkness. As the eyes and the ears are affected this is a great help and will bring relief too many sufferers.

Painkillers

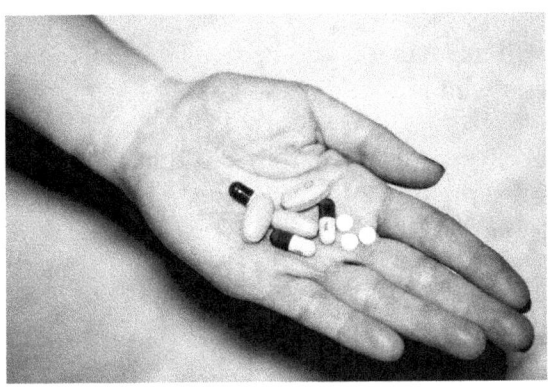

There are excellent drug cures on the market as well. There are drugs that will prevent the attack and others that will relieve the pain once it has already started. As the understanding of the disease grows the better the treatments become. They are more effective than they used to be and they are also more fast acting. It is a good thing to always give your physician feedback on any new drug he prescribes for you. This helps him or her in turn to help other patients more effectively.

There are drugs known as triptans which actually help interrupt the disease process. They will also rid you of the symptoms and either shorten the length of an attack or stop it altogether. They are not just painkillers and should therefore be taken under a medical practitioner's guidance.

There is good news for those sufferers who cannot afford these drugs. There is a triptan drug which will be going generic very soon if it has not already done so.

This will mean that it will be freely available for those sufferers who formerly could not afford to pay for it.

It is always better to take medication as soon as you feel the symptoms of migraine as opposed to waiting for the pain to set in.

There are many types of medication to abort the pain before it gets a grip on you.

If you find that the substance that your medical practitioner prescribed for you does not have the desired effect, discuss it with him and he will be able to prescribe something else that might be better for you.

All sufferers are different and what works for the one does not necessarily work for the other. Luckily there are enough types of drugs on the market for you to be able to try a few out until you get satisfaction.

Sometimes a combination of medications can have the desired effect. This must be done under the strict supervision of your medical practitioner.

It is so important to break the cycle of pain before it gets too severe otherwise you will have to wait until it works out of your system. This could take hours or in some cases even days.

There are no definite tests your doctor can do to ascertain whether or not you are a migraine sufferer. When all other possible causes for your headaches have been ruled out your doctor will assume that migraine is the problem.

It is always wise to document the drugs you have tried so that you will know which have worked for you and which perhaps had side effects or were not effective enough.

Armed with this information it is always easier to consult with the medical practitioner about your prescribed drugs and current treatment.

If you decide to discontinue a drug for any reason, let your medical practitioner know about your decision and give him the reason.

This information could help him when treating other patients as well. As there is not enough information available about this disease the more information medical practitioners can get from sufferers the more it helps them to help other sufferers.

Always remember to diarise any medication you have tried and not had good results from. Write down the date and the name of the product as this will save you the trouble of having to repeat a prescription. One does not always remember the names of all the drugs.

It is also necessary to get advice from your doctor before you use various drugs you have bought over the counter. Mixing drugs is not always a good thing and could cause complications.

Always read the labels of medication very carefully and adhere to the instructions. t is vital to take the medication as it is prescribed. Over dosing can occur when a patient becomes overwhelmed by pain.

It is wise to take soluble painkillers as they are more readily absorbed by your system and you will get the benefit of them faster.

Painkillers are also available as suppositories. These are especially good if the patient is vomiting.

Many anti migraine drugs have side effects so it is a good idea to not take them for too long a period. Try reducing the dosage when you can and then try and stop taking them altogether. It is not good to be dependant on drugs for too long. If you can do without them it will be a good thing.

Trying Better To Understand The Disease

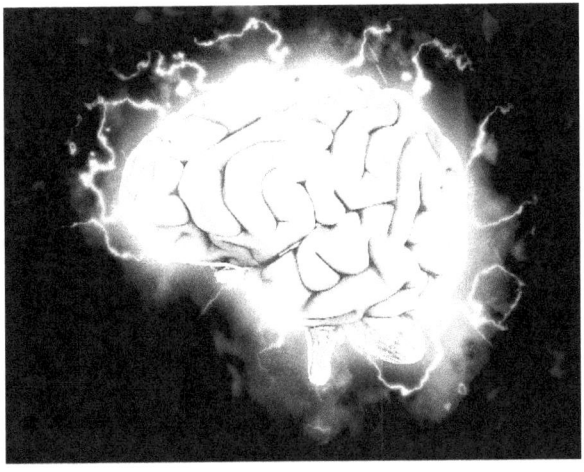

Migraine is an intense throbbing pain on one side of the head. It can occur on either side or in front of the head.

It is a good idea to get as much knowledge of the disease as possible as there is not very much information to be had on the subject. As medical science has not yet proved what it is exactly that causes the disease it is a good idea to exchange notes with someone you know who is also a sufferer of the disease.

By comparing symptoms and treatments you get a broader view of migraine. When you understand what is causing the pain it makes it easier for you to be able to manage the attacks.

Various factors can trigger off an attack. Stress, over tiredness, anxiety, diet, caffeine or in women it could be hormonal changes.

For regular sufferers it could be advantageous to keep a diary of migraine attacks. This could show a pattern of frequency and what triggers off the attacks.

You could in this way spot what it is that is triggering your attacks and avoid the situations in the future. It could be stress or something in your diet. By regularly documenting the day and time when each attack started, how you were feeling at the time and what you ate could be vital clues to what is causing your attacks.

You would then be able to ward off future attacks by eliminating certain foods from your diet or not getting stressed or avoiding certain situations that you know will cause you anxiety or restlessness.

This is something that no one else can do for you and to avoid having the invasion of this disease in your life make the effort of playing a part in finding relief.

What is the cause of the headache? You might wonder why your head gets so intensely sore. The skull can not feel pain but there is a network of nerves covering the scalp and some of them extend into the face which can feel pain.

The ends of these nerves can be stimulated by various factors such as stress and muscular tension.

Here is an example of someone who had very frequent migraine attacks and did not realise immediately what was triggering them off Kevin, who suffered from sever migraine for many years realised that motoring home from work everyday he would be facing the sun. Inadvertently a ray of sunshine would be reflected on a vehicle in front of him or on some other object.

Just for a split second his eyes would catch the flickering light and this would be enough to trigger off a migraine attack.

By never motoring during the daytime without wearing his prescription sun glasses he could ward off numerous attacks. Sometimes it is just a small adjustment you need to make in order to prevent an attack being triggered off.

It is always good to be proactive and to avoid situations that you know will leave you with this excruciating pain.

Even if you are not a migraine sufferer yourself your quality of life can be affected by the disease if you live with a family member or members that suffer from this disease.

It always rears its ugly head when you least expect it. It is sometimes difficult for family members to have plans disrupted because one of the members has an attack. One has to learn sympathy for this disease and realise that they have no control over the time the attack starts.

When you are in this state you do not feel like going out and having fun. The only thought in your mind is to get rid of the pain. You have to retreat to a dark room where you can rest with no noise or disturbances.

It is good to educate the children about migraine if one of the parents is suffering from the disease. If they realise that this is a disease and not an excuse for the parent to get out of taking them somewhere or trying to opt out of any other duty they will not put unnecessary pressure on the sufferer.

It might be a good idea to educate your employer and co workers about the disease as well so that they will realise that it is a neurological disease and not something you pretend to be having in order to shirk your duties.

Unfortunately there is not enough knowledge and awareness of this disease among the general public. Many people still think that migraine is just another headache and will think that those who suffer from it are over reacting or putting on about the severity of the pain.

How Can You Improve Your Quality Of Life?

The more information you can gather about your disease the better you will understand the condition. It is one of the most misunderstood diseases. Many people think that it is just another headache with a fancy name that only women get. There are support groups that share information with sufferers and supply information to health carers. There is satisfaction in knowing that you are not alone.

These migraine associations are busy increasing the awareness of the disease to the public and this in turn will stimulate the medical profession to do more research on the subject.

This condition should not just be put down to a debilitating headache but should be regarded more seriously. It is a disruptive and disabling disease for those who suffer regularly from it. Once family and friends realise that this is a real disease they will have more sympathy and support for your condition.

Educate your immediate family and friends about the disease so that if you have to unexpectedly cancel plans because of an attack they will understand that you are not merely using a headache as an excuse.

The general public need to understand that this is a disease and can attack at any time of the day or night.

You can play your part by contributing information you might have learnt through your own experience. By sharing information researchers can put together a better picture of what sufferers go through and this could be the breakthrough they need to find out more about the disease.

In knowledge there is always strength. One always feels better about a problem when you have some knowledge of what is going on. This will help you better to manage migraine.

The more people know about the disease the easier it will be for them to expect better medical care from practitioners.

The impact of this disease on any country's economy is enormous considering

how many people take off sick leave per annum due to this condition. It is becoming as common as influenza as more and more people become prone to migraine attacks.

It is impossible to function in any type of job when you are going through an attack. Your mind cannot function correctly and many people have such pain in their eyes that they cannot go into the light.

There is only one course of action to take and that is to stay at home in a quiet darkened room and wait for the attack to subside.

Eat a healthy diet and take food supplements. They are freely available in health stores and many other stores. These will help combat fatigue and drop in blood sugar when you inadvertently miss meals.

Exercise is so important. Have a healthy exercise routine but do not partake in any strenuous sport where a sudden bump or jolt could trigger off a migraine attack.

If stress and anxiety are your problems attend relaxation classes and learn how to handle yourself when you get into this state. By learning to relax you will feel the benefits and could possibly ward off many attacks of migraine.

Get plenty of fresh air. Quite often sufferers begin to feel "fuzzy" in their heads when they are in a closed environment for a time. This can in turn trigger off a headache.

Keep out of areas where there is cigarette smoke. This can also be a triggering factor for migraine sufferers. Healthy living is already a step nearer to solving your problem.

You might not be able to completely cure migraine but you can give yourself a better quality of life by minimising the amount of attacks you have.

The fact that the sufferer is literally disabled for a number of hours or days by intense pain with symptoms like partial blindness and deafness and numbness in the limbs makes it a very real disease.

When young children suffer from this disease it is good to remember that they are suffering pain and if they are unmanageable for a few hours one has to be sympathetic.

Most children normally experience the pain in the abdominal region and this can be very distressing for them. In severe cases this could last up to 72 hours.

If you are on prescribed drugs you must take them as directed by the medical practitioner. Notify him immediately if you experience any side effects.

Who Does Migraine Affect Most?

As migraine is a common disease most people will at some time or another experience an attack. It may just be one attack in a life time or it could become a regular occurrence. Migraines affect about 15% of the population.

Many people refer to any headache as a migraine. This is not so and you can have just a headache from stress or from a bump or something else. All headaches are not migraine.

This disease attacks many more women than men. Statistics show that 2 in 4 women will be sufferers and men only 1 in 12.

This disease can occur at any age, but mostly occurs in people between the ages of 10 and 40. It tends to ease off after this age and becomes less as the sufferer gets older. This is not always the case as there are older sufferers who still experience attacks of migraine.

This disease affects young children as well as adults. They often start migraine headaches when they are young or they could only begin when they reach adolescence. Fortunately it seems that children who suffer from migraine tend to grow out of the disease. There is no known fact why this occurs but it is a fortunate state of affairs.

The fact that more women than men are sufferers could be put down to the fact that many women's hormonal changes are also causes of this disease. Hormone therapy could be beneficial to some of these women. Speak to your medical practitioner about it.

It does appear to be a fact that these women will have less or no headaches after they have reached menopause.

It could be that women experience more stress than men due to the complexity of their careers and homemaking and parenting responsibilities.

It does appear to be a fact that this disease runs in families which would mean that it could be genetically transmitted. It could be that the factors that trigger off the disease are genetically transmitted rather than the disease itself.

The general economy is also affected by this disease with the loss of productivity. It costs employers millions of dollars per annum when they have staff members who need to frequently have time off. There is no way a sufferer can cope with a job during an attack.

It also makes an enormous impact on any countries health and medical resources. Research is also an ongoing project which costs a lot of money. The cost to the individuals for over the counter drugs is also astronomical.

Employers could try and give migraine sufferers on their staff more flexible hours so that they do not become over tired or stressed. This could possible reduce attacks and the employer would benefit by it.

General Factors That Could Trigger Off An Attack

According to data collected from studies of various cases it appears that there are a number of factors that can trigger a migraine attack. This information was gathered over time with various groups of migraine sufferers.

It appears that there is no evidence to prove that these substances and conditions do trigger off an attack.

By comparing notes with various sufferers one can come to the conclusion that these factors do have an influence on this disease and by keeping a record of your own attacks you will with time be able to realise what is affecting you adversely.

Prevention is better than cure – so if you can prevent these attacks by watching your diet or stress levels it could be very advantageous for you.

Stress And Any Form Of Anxiety

This is probably one of the most important factors in triggering off a migraine. Many migraine sufferers clench or grind their teeth in their sleep and this could

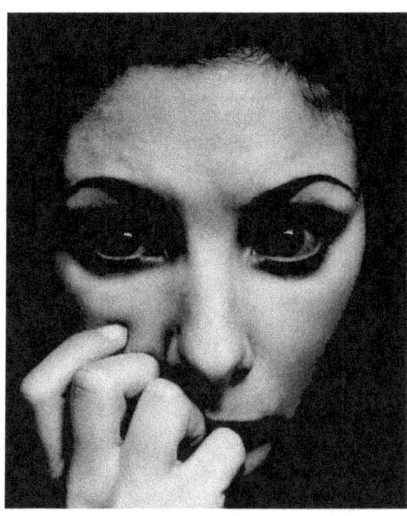

trigger off an attack. A device can be made by a dentist to cover the front teeth at night so that the grinding cannot take place. This will reduce pain in the jaw and could be a factor to reduce migraine attacks.

Post Stress

The attack could occur after the stress is over. This is why many sufferers have attacks once they begin to relax, for example when they are on vacation or over a weekend.

Bright Lights And Flickering Lights

You do not have to be exposed to bright or flickering lights for long before you will find that your eyes begin to ache and you will feel the symptoms of the headache starting.

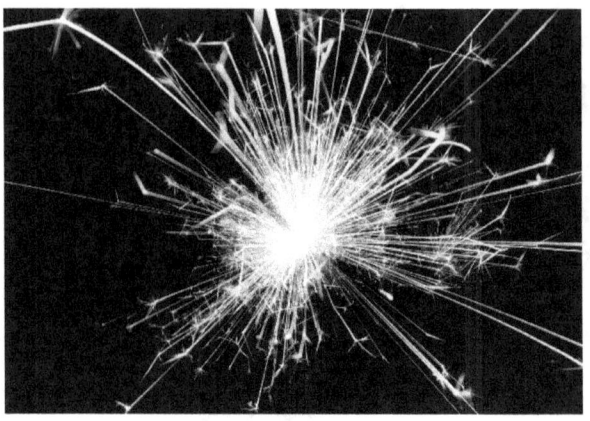

Dehydration

This is an important factor and doctors are realising that this could trigger off many sufferers migraine.

Loud Noises

This factor seems to be particularly true when the sufferer is over tired or anxious.

Lack Of Sleep Or Any Change In Your Sleep Pattern

This can cause stress and in turn this will cause an attack.

Alcohol

Moderation in the intake of alcohol is recommended.

Caffeine

Caffeine is not recommended and yet there are sufferers who have reported that by drinking a cup of coffee when they feel the onslaught of an attack they can actually ward it off. There are certain prescription drugs that contain caffeine which have

proved to be beneficial for severe attacks of migraine. You will have to decide for yourself how this substance reacts with your condition. If you are addicted to caffeine and you suddenly stop taking it, it could cause you to have a migraine attack.

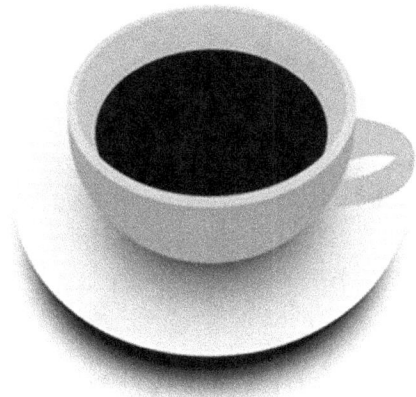

Menstrual Cycle In Women Or The Use Of Contraceptive Pills

This can be due to estrogen levels dropping at this time.

Certain Allergies

Certain allergies could trigger a migraine.

Smoking Or The Exposure To Smoke

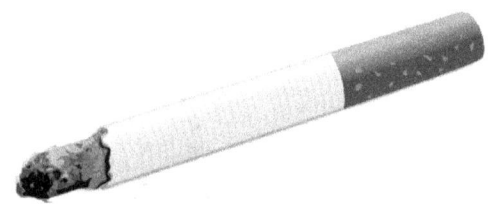

It is advisable to stop smoking if you are a smoker and avoid areas where you will be exposed to smoke even for a little while.

Skipping Meals

This is a huge factor as the blood sugar can drop too low. It is a good idea to take food supplements and this does help sustain the body if you have to skip a meal

Being Over Tired

This causes stress.

Various Types Of Food

In this category many types of food have been mentioned. There is little or no evidence to prove that chocolate, cheese and red wine. Smoked fish and peanut butter and various fruits were also named as causes of migraine. There is no evidence that any of these food types are the cause of migraine although many sufferers do name them as culprits.

Various Types Of Odors And Perfumes

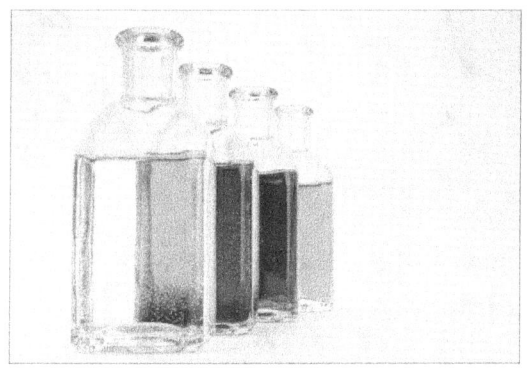

Changes In The Weather

This factor was also named by some candidates of research groups as a possible trigger for their attacks. There is no scientific proof for this but many people do experience migraine when the weather changes. Many sufferers find that when it is windy they are more prone to an attack.

Weather Change

As opposed to seasonal change, weather change was named as being a factor especially in high humidity with plus high or low temperatures.

Change In Altitude

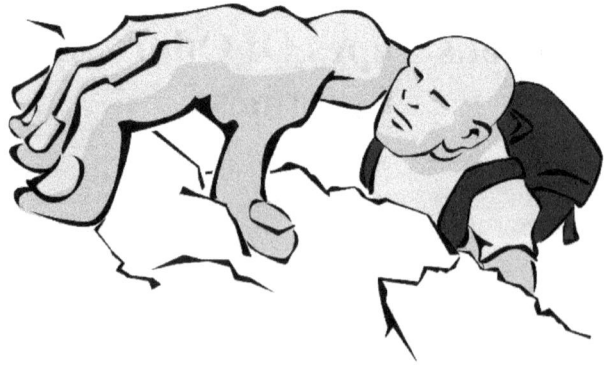

This could also be a factor in causing a migraine.

Lack Of Exercise

This could also be a contributing factor.

Bottling Up Your Emotions

This can be very bad for you as when you eventually "explode" you will inevitably end up with a headache. Avoid situations where you will be tempted to lose your temper.

Preservatives And Additives In Food

An allergy to these substances could trigger off a migraine attack. Make a note of this in your migraine diary so that you will be aware of the fact when you ate something containing additives.

Prescribed Spectacles

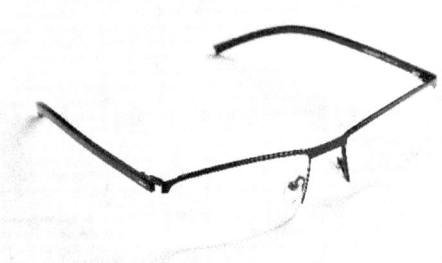

It is thought that spectacles that are not correctly prescribed could trigger off migraine. Make sure that you are wearing spectacles that suit your eyes if not have your eyes retested and get a pair that are right for your eyes as this could be the cause of your headaches.

Migraine sufferers should do their best to identify the factors that trigger off their individual attacks. If you know what is triggering off the attack you can avoid the situation at all costs.

It could be you need to change your diet or avoid skipping meals. Changing your sleep pattern might help. Moderation is all things are a good habit. Maybe you could cut down on your alcohol and caffeine intake and avoid places where there are very bright, flickering lights and very loud noises.

You might need to cut down on stress and try and be more relaxed. Avoid situations that will make you lose your temper or get over anxious.

Make an effort to make a study of what triggers off your attacks and you will be able to live a better quality of life.

Types Of Headaches

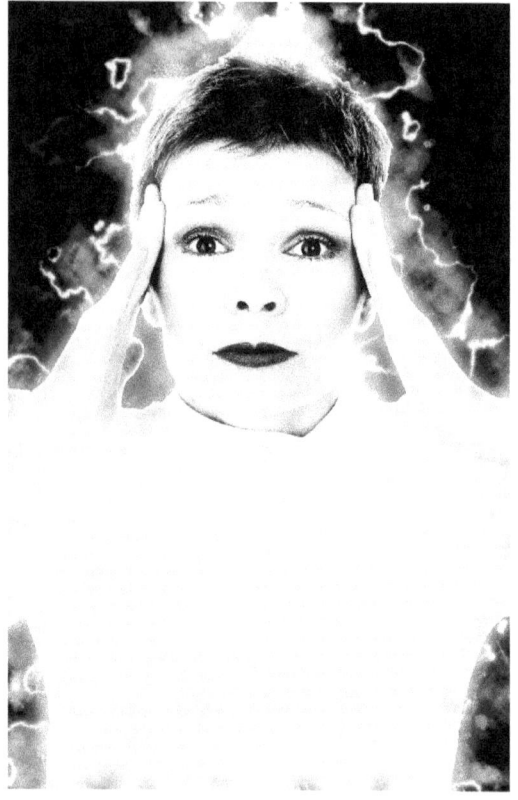

Many people assume that they have a migraine when they get a headache. This is not the case as migraine is completely something different to the usual headache.

If you have persistent headaches they obviously must have a cause and it is advisable to seek medical help in ascertaining what the cause is.

There are headaches caused by sinus problems. This is caused by pressure as a result of blocked sinuses.

Consult a doctor to make sure that this is the case and he or she will be able to treat you.

Tension headaches are very common among adults. This is normally due to the daily stresses that we have to deal with in modern living. This normally feels like there is a band applying pressure to the head. These headaches could last a few minutes or longer depending on how long the stress prevails.

Usually the pain can be alleviated by relaxing with your eyes closed for a while and thinking of something other than what caused the stress.

By doing some activity like sport or gardening the tension will subside and the pain will be gone. These headaches can more or less be controlled by the sufferer.

There are headaches that are caused by a lack of sleep or over indulgence in alcohol.

A headache could be caused by taking an overdose of painkillers or some other substance. It is always wise to read the label of medication containers very well and adhere to the instructions given.

There are women who suffer from menstrual headaches. These often lead to migraine. This is believed to be related to the fact that the estrogen levels change during the menstrual cycle.

Women are often accused of "putting on a headache" but these migraine attacks are very real and could put the sufferer out of action for a number of hours or even days.

There is a type of headache know as a cluster headache. This type of headache recurs over a period of time and can cause a lot of pain. These headaches can become very severe and will become more painful than migraine in many cases.

They occur in clusters mostly at the same time of the day. This could carry on for several weeks. The pain is very severe and other symptoms are nausea, sensitivity to light and the eye and nose on the affected sod of the face could become swollen and red. The sufferers report feeling very restless and agitated.

It appears to attack more men than women in the age group between 20 and 50 years of age.

Medical practitioners will subscribe drugs for the severe pain either orally, injection or a nasal spray. There are drugs available to suppress future attacks.

Migraine is not specifically a type of headache.

Headaches are just one of the symptoms of the disease. There are many others which vary from partial blindness and deafness to numbness in the hands and arms. The face can also go partially numb as well as the lips and tongue in some patients. Speech can be slurred and a dull feeling can occur in the head.

There are various other symptoms that sufferers can experience. Not all attacks will be the same. This is a disabling disease and can attack at any time.

Conclusion

Once you have positively been diagnosed with migraine do not see it as a life sentence. It can be managed.

Diarise all the data just prior to an attack, food types and emotional state. By regularly doing this you will be able to see a pattern of events emerging. You can then start eliminating food types one by one and you will eventually realise what food types are detrimental to you if that is the cause of migraine.

Emotional pattern is easier to discern. You will then be able to train yourself not to get over tired or stressed. Letting go of your anger versus bottling up your emotions could be the answer.

You might be a sufferer who has the attacks triggered off by flashing or flickering lights or loud noises. You can then do your best to avoid these situations.

Being aware of what triggers off attacks will make it easier to manage the disease and the attacks will become less frequent.

Medical science is constantly improving and finding out new cures for migraine so there is always hope that they will come up with something that could cure you completely.

I hope that my studies have benefited you and your family and that you will find relief from this painful and frustrating disease.